Cancer Ain't Cute!

Jeanetta Bryant

ISBN: 978-1-954529-35-9

Published by PlayPen Publishing

www.playpenpublishing.com

Ellenwood, GA USA

I want to dedicate this book to my two wonderful boys, Brayden and Bryce. Everything I do, I do with your well-being in heart. I sincerely hope that I have made you proud, and that you both know how much I love you.

~Mommy

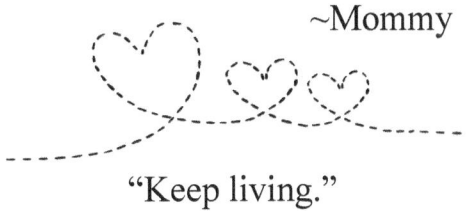

"Keep living."

"It will be greater later."

~Mama

Have a seat. Let me tell you something.

I want to take you on a journey through my cancer experience. I want to offer an unfiltered and honest version of what cancer looks like and share insights that are often not discussed. I acknowledge that cancer is not a cute experience, but I would like to offer hope by sharing how it is possible to come out on the other side and find something even more beautiful than before.

I want to take you down my road and let you see what they DON'T tell you.

Let's prepare ourselves for this journey, as the road ahead has numerous potholes, sinkholes, and sewage. Despite all of this, let's stay strong and continue moving forward together. We will eventually reach the end of the street, and when we do, you will realize how much you have accomplished. You will look back and say to yourself, "My God, how did you carry me down this ugly road, and I come out on the other side not looking like what I have been through?" This realization will be a testament to your strength, and you will know that you have done a job well done. During my journey, I faced the loss of many things that I believed defined me, such as my hair, waistline, nails, and money. However, I learned that God promised his children healing, redemption, and renewal in our lives. With unwavering faith in God, I confidently trusted that he would restore what I had lost and even increase all future blessing. This promise from God inspired me to keep going, knowing I would someday reap a harvest.

The Road to Recovery: A Message of Perseverance and Faith

I remember my oncologist saying, "We can stop now. I think you've had enough." I looked at him and said, "NO! The science says that I'm supposed to have 16 rounds of chemo. I'm not stopping. I'm going to do my 16 rounds of chemo because I do not want a single chance of this cancer coming back!"

Recovery isn't always pretty, but it's a journey worth taking. As my mama used to say, "Keep living." I fought hard for my life and realized God had my back. Nothing in life happens without God's permission, and Satan couldn't touch me. God had faith in me and knew I wouldn't curse Him or falter in my faith. Despite my afflictions, I emerged victorious and unbreakable like never before. God bet on me. *God told him to go ahead and try her because I know my child. She will never curse me and die. Go ahead, try her, but let me tell you this much: when you try her, you can't lay a finger on her, and you can't kill her.* That's what my God told Satan about me. *Go ahead*, and this affliction of stage 3 breast cancer was placed upon me. God went before me and told Satan, *You can't kill her!* I'm standing! I'm still here!

I remember a time when the chemo became too much for me to bear. My swelling was so severe in my arms, hands, legs, and feet. I was carrying around at least 15 pounds of fluid, and towards the end of chemo, I was gaining 2-3 pounds per week. You could see the sock wording imprinted on my skin. The swelling caused my skin to get fire-hot, red, itchy, and sensitive to the touch. The fluid caused my joints to ache. Walking was damn near unbearable due to the massive amount of fluid and weight gain. On days that I wanted to give up, all I could hear in my head was my mama's voice from when I was a small child. When I went through tough times as a kid, my mama always reminded me, "It gets greater later." So, I knew I had to stay the course.

I felt as though my doctor saw the suffering in me. It was as though he was telling me to stop fighting, curse God, and die. At least that's how I felt! How could I receive blessings from the Lord and not be able to deal with the pain and suffering? For me, my blessing was to be told that I was cancer-free. I had to go through the pain and suffering that I endured. This is what I mean when I say cancer ain't cute. Nothing about this journey was pretty, but I went through it, and now I'm on my way to the other side. I'm ready to receive my blessings from the Lord because I stayed the course. I was chosen. I was cherry-picked to go through this. So, I took my diagnosis like a woman; I cried; I had sleepless nights. I had pain going through my body, and every time I wanted to give up, I reminded myself that He picked one of his baddest, strongest warriors out there to fight this fight. You got this! Everybody cannot carry this cross on their back, but you can. Bravely, I carried that cross with grace, dignity, integrity, and ...

HERE I AM!

TABLE OF CONTENTS

Introduction: The Road to Recovery: A Message of Perseverance and Faith — VI

Chapter ONE: The Beginning — 1

Chapter TWO: The Shower — 9

Chapter THREE: Tiny Intruder — 13

Chapter FOUR: Biopsy Day — 17

Chapter FIVE: The Red Devil — 25

Chapter SIX: Can A Sista Get A Break? — 31

Chapter SEVEN: A New Normal That Nobody Asked For! — 39

A Letter To My Boys — 43

CANCER AIN'T CUTE!

Chapter ONE

The Beginning

"Our Father, who art in heaven, hallowed be thy name; thy kingdom come; thy will be done; on earth as it is in heaven. Give us this day our daily bread. And forgive us our trespasses, as we forgive those who trespass against us. And lead us not into temptation; but deliver us from the evil one. For thine is the kingdom, the power and the glory, for ever and ever. Amen." Luke (11:2-4)

A nurse, covered from head to toe in PPE, walked into the room. She was holding a silver tray of meds that almost looked like cocktails should have been placed on it. She approached me with an IV bag inside a light-protected bag. I looked at her like *What are you about to do with that*, and *Why do you have on this gown, face mask, and long gloves covering your gown?* She said, "We have to wear this protective gear when we administer the chemo to you. It can't touch our skin because it will make us sick." I was in disbelief at how a drug that was this dangerous to even handle was deemed okay to go into my body, though? Right then, it hit me that I was SICK, and I was about to be in a fight for my life. My life, as I knew it, would never be the same. I sat there for hours as the toxic and potentially lethal drug, drip and drip and dripped into my port. It was the longest four hours of my life! I asked myself, *What is happening to me? God, where are you?* As I sat there, I wanted to pray but I couldn't come up with my own words. This small voice in my head told me when you can't pray, just say the Lord's prayer. So, I sat still as this chemo was slowly dripping into my port. I closed my eyes and started reciting the Lord's prayer.

Who's Jeanetta "Star Baby" Bryant?

Both names hold a significant place in my life, and I always felt the need to live up to both names and their meanings. Being the youngest, you can imagine I was all over the place. I acted in the school plays, sang, danced, and was a cheerleader and a straight-up go-getter. I did everything that could be done as a child. I loved life and was treated and acted like a little STAR in my family. While in school, I would often say to myself, *None of this crap they are talking about is essential. Who cares what side I stapled my paper on? Who cares about the ink spot on my paper? Who cares who won the Super Bowl?* That was how I thought back then. I would ask my teachers, "Do you know there's someone out there right now being told they might not make it in the next 24 hours? Do you know right now, someone is being told they have a disease that is going to kill them, and you are tripping about the trivial stuff?" That's how my mind worked; I didn't know that my passion would turn my life into a life of service to others.

That was when my dream of becoming a nurse was born. And for 25 years, I have been chasing that dream. I want to live a life of service to help others, give of myself, and ensure that someone else is okay. But life sure does have a funny way of telling you to hold up and wait a minute. It's not your time. When life did that to me, my faith in God was tested. I felt like I gave everyone else their heart's desires, but why couldn't He grant me the desires of my heart? Then, I started questioning myself and my decisions after every setback and moment of disappointment from a lousy job and relationship choices. That spark and light started to dim in my eyes, and I became complacent.

As I became an adult, I transitioned into my role of Jeanetta, which my life then started to fashion itself after my namesake. I started being the glue that held what family members were left together. I started hosting all of the holiday events at my home. I started being the caregiver to my mom and the emotional support to a few family members and friends. I became a nurturing woman and took care of everyone around me. I made sure that everyone with me was good. The more my plate filled up with people's needs and desires, the less space there was for me. And in typical Jeanetta fashion, I allowed everyone's issues to pile up on my plate.

I married my first husband and had my eldest son with him. However, that marriage was merely a test run. We stayed together for eight years but were only married for six months. My husband, who was supposedly a God-fearing man, was always at the church before the doors even opened and stayed until they turned the lights off. While he was busy with the church, I deepened my faith and learned a lot about God's grace and mercy. But, I always felt like something was off. Despite his claims of being a God-fearing man, his actions as a husband were mediocre, and I felt like I wasn't getting the love and respect I deserved. In the end, I realized he was not the man for me.

Eventually, I realized that this marriage had become toxic and was causing harm to my spirituality, mind, heart, and self-worth. So, I decided to end it and start a new life for myself and my son. However, it took me five years to obtain a divorce. During this time, some wonderful people came into my life: Treanda, Ivy, Johanna, and Brittney. These women became the backbone I needed to face the many challenges ahead

Ivy, Treanda, and Johanna were women that I worked with for a few years. We developed a bond that has carried us for many years. We spent holidays, weekends, and birthdays together. During my darkest hours, they became family to my son Brayden, and their kids became cousins to him. They became my sisters-in-Christ. There was never a time that I couldn't call on them for a word of encouragement or prayer. Life eventually became stable, and I was content being a single mom. I had my girlfriends, and that's all I thought I needed. As anyone who has been through a divorce, it was very taxing dealing with the anxiety from the pending court dates, constant rescheduling, lies, and mud-slinging. You name it, those five years were unimaginable!

During those years, it was tough for me to pray. I felt like God had abandoned me and that he no longer heard my cries. I was churched out and genuinely felt like I had nowhere to turn. My life was at work, at home, watching DVDs with Brayden, and that's it.

One night, a girlfriend invited me to this bar for dinner and drinks. I was so reluctant to go, but I could easily say yes after a few glasses of red wine. To my surprise, this night would be the night that I would meet the man created just for me. Years later, this man would be the one to help me walk, hold me up to rub my back, kiss my scars, wipe my tears away, and pray for me. This man would stand before me and take some of the blows I would soon face eight years later. That night, I met my husband, provider, protector, first responder, and youngest son's dad, Bryan.

From the moment we started dating, Bryan always had my back. He was there to save and support me whenever I faced life's challenges. I, in turn, provided him with the nurturing support he needed during his own difficult breakup. We were each other's rock, and I felt like I was on top of the world with him by my side. I knew that God had brought us together for a reason, and I was grateful for every moment we spent together. When we first started dating, my partner was always there for me whenever I needed saving or support. In particular, he stood by my side when I was going through my divorce and never showed any moments of intimidation during the process. He was very confident in his ability to love and care for me. Likewise, I provided him with the nurturing support he needed as he was also going through a difficult breakup. We were each other's peace, and I was so happy to finally find someone who was such a positive force in my life. For once, I felt like I was on top of the world, and I knew that God had brought this man into my life for a reason.

After eight long years, I finally realized why certain people had come into my life and why some had left. Looking back, it's clear that God had a plan for me all along, and these people were meant to guide me through my journey. Even though it may have been tough at times, I wouldn't change a thing. Now, I have a supportive team, a loving family, and a life for which I'm grateful. It's amazing how everything comes full circle when we trust the journey.

How did Star Baby go from being born in Grady Memorial Hospital to being a Cancer patient?

I was born and raised in Atlanta, GA. I am a "Grady Baby," as we originals born at Grady Memorial Hospital call ourselves. I was the last of 13 grandchildren to be born into my family, and because of that, my grandmother's name, Jeanetta, was bestowed upon me. I have always been proud of my name. My grandmother was a strong vibration and larger-than-life figure in our family. On top of carrying my grandmother's name and being the youngest of a large family, my father also gave me a name more prominent than life itself. He gave me the nickname Star Baby. He said he saw stars in my eyes the day I was born, which I would joke about. I thought it was lame. I told him, "Daddy, those were not stars you saw in my eyes. Those were the lights from the delivery room." He and I always laughed about this; it was our little thing. I didn't understand why I was chosen to carry both names back then. I always felt differently about life and how I viewed it, but I couldn't put my finger on it. I would soon find out what all of this was going to mean. I did not know that the lesson on my names I carried around would strengthen me after learning there was a possibility of losing the life I valued and loved.

90 Days In

In a mere 90 days, everything that defined me was lost. My hair, breasts, nails, toenails, femininity, mind, and body vanished in an instant. All due to a seemingly insignificant lump in my breast? This microscopic growth had the power to devastate my life, relationships, finances, and even my marriage if I allowed it. The intense rage that ensued was overwhelming. It pushed me into a dark abyss with no escape. But I refused to succumb to this monster. I channeled the anger and transformed it into a fierce determination to battle for my life, which was hanging in the balance. Because one thing is true, "Cancer ain't cute, and this is what they don't tell you." Feeling yourself burning from the inside out, drives you into a mental state of hell on Earth. After chemo, I laid in bed, propped my legs up on pillows, curled my toes, and felt my fingernails and toenails burning. They felt like they were detaching from my nail beds until they eventually turned black and fell off! It was nearly impossible to open cans and even pull my pants up. I had to figure out ways to improvise my basic everyday processes. I couldn't stand to wear shoes, and Crocs™ became my saving grace for work. Three months ... that's all it took to lose what made me ... ME!

I remember my scalp would hurt, ache, and burn in patches until it ultimately started to fall out. But no one tells you this. I would lay there and ask God, *What did I do in my life to deserve this? Who have I upset? God, I haven't been perfect, but I haven't been all that bad either.* I was so upset with God that I didn't see the bigger picture at the time. All I saw was how I had worshiped myself and my looks over God. But again, this is not something they show you because all they show is the commercial side of cancer.

Pink

Before I was diagnosed with breast cancer, I was familiar with what we all see every October about it. Pink ribbons, pink pom poms, T-shirts, and smiling, happy, bald women walking for the cure made it look like we all wanted to be a part of this. For one month out of a year, we are bombarded with ads during prime-time football games about "breast cancer awareness," but honestly, what does awareness look like?

Calm Before The Storm

Cancer took everything from me but my life. I could barely take care of my kids due to the indescribable level of pain in my body and fatigue. The amount of fluid that was building up in my body due to the chemo made it challenging to walk and breathe. I developed lymphedema in my arm and axillary web syndrome (cording). All of this, combined with what was mentally going on with me, left me feeling unattractive and useless. I felt like a financial burden to my husband. Not being able to help him with the bills made me feel like I was a financial burden to him. I couldn't keep up my house or cook for my kids; this made me feel like I was failing as a wife and a mother. My income was cut in half, and he was away from home more to make ends meet for the family. Cancer overall caused a cluster of crap in my life in just a matter of months, and that's going to take years to recover from. But, this is what they don't tell you. Mainstream media makes this look like a thing you go through where your hair falls out, and at the end, you get to have a big parade where you get to wear all pink with your supporters. What they don't show you is the raw, unedited version of the unprecedented toll cancer takes on your life.

Let's journey back six months before a tiny intruder decided to take up residence in my body. Surrounded by a loving group of colleagues, I was a happy-go-lucky worker who had been perfecting my craft for years. One of my besties was a mammogram technician, and we shared a special bond because we worked in the same building. I was a social butterfly, fluttering between parties and gatherings, and my husband and I had just moved into our new nest, which I loved to entertain in and decorate. Our home was full of family and friends. Life was blissful as a newlywed, and my sons kept me giggling all day long. I lovingly call them "Tom and Jerry."

Life was like a dream come true! I got accepted into the nursing program at Chamberlin University, which was set to kick off in January 2023. My career was soaring high, but I wanted more. So, I landed a new gig, and it felt like I was on top of the world! I took a break from work to enjoy Christmas with my family in our new home, and it was pure magic. The sweet smell of cinnamon spice filled the air, and everything was merry and bright. But, as fate would have it, one Sunday evening changed everything.

Chapter TWO

The Shower

I will sprinkle clean water on you, and you will be clean; I will cleanse you from all your impurities and from all your idols. -Ezekiel (36:25)

I began my regular shower routine, where I washed my hair and my entire body. Back then, I used to have truly large breasts; I would have to pick them up to wash underneath. This particular night, I'm doing my thing, and I go to lift my breast to clean underneath it. Stay with me. I lifted my breast; I didn't press it or probe it; nothing. I merely lifted it, and that's it. As I lifted my breast, I felt this small cluster of what felt like tiny stones in my breast. Immediately, shock waves, nerves, and anxiety flooded over me.

I could barely finish my shower! So I jumped out, took a deep breath, and said, "Lord, please don't let this be." I looked into the mirror and didn't see anything at first glance. Then, I remembered hearing all the press about placing your hands on your hips and looking at your breasts to see if they were the same size. Then, raise your hands above your head to see if there was any dimpling. Suddenly, I saw that dimpling in my breast. It looked like someone had placed their thumb in some dough and left an indention in my left nipple area. That moment was the first time I saw my soul leave my body because I felt the truth in my heart. All I could do was stand there and look at myself just as bare as I came into this world. I was afraid to step out of this bathroom to tell my husband of a year and a half that I found lumps in my breast.

With tears in my eyes, I walked out of the bathroom, and my face was lifeless. Bryan asked me, "Babe, what's going on?" I couldn't speak, so he asked me again, but I still couldn't talk. The third time, he stood up, walked towards me, and asked me again. All I could do was fall into his arms. At that moment, I told him that I felt something in my breast. He looked me in my eyes and said in the sweetest, calmest, secure voice, "Okay, babe, we got this. Let's find out what this is before you freak out." I let him feel it at least twenty-five times that night, took eight other pictures, and sent the photos to a few of my girls working in healthcare. After I sent all these boob shoots to my girls, Ivy picked up the phone and called me and said we are going to get you an appointment tonight. She made a call to the company that I hadn't worked for in over eight years. We still had a mutual friend, Tre, who worked in the women's mammogram department. When I tell you, those women interceded on my behalf on that Sunday night, January 8th! They set me up to get a mammogram on Tuesday morning without seeing a doctor first. Remember, now that I had no insurance and had just started my new job five days prior.

Monday Morning

Let's fast forward to Monday morning. I was clearly running on nothing but fumes. In an effort to put on a happy face and learn my new position, I quickly chugged a few Red Bulls™. Despite my best efforts, my trainer could tell I was deeply struggling. My bloodshot eyes and numb demeanor gave it away. I was just numb, and she asked me if I was okay. At that moment, I broke, and the tears started to flow. She invited me into a private patient room to talk.

When we walked into the room, I began to tell her about what I had discovered the night before. In a frantic moment of desperation, I asked her if she wanted to see my breast. She was a little taken aback by this, but she agreed because she is a woman and medical professional. After I asked, I thought to myself, *Girl, what have you just done? You just asked this lady you hardly know to touch your breast?* While probing, she tried to comfort me by suggesting other possible things that the cluster could be. She even shared her story about her breast health again to help calm me down. It was time to return to work right after my appointment, and I had to make good on their investment. I was a new hire, so get out there and work!

Luckily, I was in training then, so I didn't have to deal with people face-to-face. Still, it looked like a black cloud was hanging over me to the team. I can assure you they were looking like, *what's wrong with the new girl? She looks a mess.* I was doing a lot of computer training while learning the system and all the ins and outs of this new place. As I tried to focus and ignore this unfamiliar object in my body, my phone continuously buzzed with reminders of my upcoming appointment the following day. I hadn't mentioned any of this to my new manager yet. I was fortunate to have a woman as my boss and a colleague who was a breast cancer survivor. She had just returned from treatment two months before they hired me, so I felt like I was in the right place at the right time. Fast forward to Tuesday, the day of my mammogram ultrasound appointment. I was anxious about the test and worried they might reject me because I didn't have insurance. I couldn't help but reminisce about the tactics my friends used to get my appointment scheduled so quickly. I anticipated something would go wrong, but fortunately, checking in for the appointment was smooth sailing. It was a huge relief.

Chapter THREE

Tiny Intruder

The journey of a thousand miles begins with one step.
-Lao Tzu

I was off to the mammogram area to change clothes, and to my surprise, my husband couldn't come to the sub-waiting area with me. I am alone again, and I badly needed to just lay on him and wait to be called back. But at that moment, it started to hit me, *When you are faced with life-altering issues, it is just you and you alone. No one can walk this walk with you but YOU!*

It made me reflect upon all the times I had given my all, even when I didn't have the energy or the wherewithal to do for others. There I was on that table alone, dealing with what life dealt me when I should have practiced more self-care. I was lying there wondering, *Is it too late? What have you done to yourself? Why didn't you take time for yourself? Now, look at you about to stroke out in this room.* Blood pressure was through the roof! When the nurse took my vitals, my pressure and heart rate were so high they threatened not to do that exam. I was sitting in that triage room with the nurse, begging her to please do this exam on me. I told her, "My blood pressure is high because I'm worried about getting the test done. If you do the test, my pressure will go down." The nurse went down the hall to speak with the tech. She got the okay to send me back only after I sat there for two hours past my original appointment time. My pressure wasn't completely lowered after taking a fast-acting blood pressure pill and two Xanax. Still, I was no longer at stoke level. So, they allowed me to go in for the mammogram.

When I walked into that room, I swear everything was moving in slow motion. The room was cold and very dark. It seemed like the nurse was talking to me underwater; I couldn't even process her words. She had me take my pink robe off and step up to the mammogram machine. That machine was so big and cold and scary to me at that moment. I swear I felt like I was walking up to the electric chair. She had me put the lumpy breast in first. She told me to take a deep breath and hold it, and the procedure began. Please remember that I am a medical professional and have worked in several areas of medicine. One of my closest girlfriends, Mel, is a mammogram tech. I have been in the room and helped Mel work with women to get set up for their mammograms. So, I know the body language of the medical staff when something is wrong. So, as this tech was doing my exam, she kept referencing how she needed to get up under my armpit. Then she stepped out of the room and told me I needed to go and get an ultrasound immediately.

At this point in my mind, there was nothing more they needed to tell me. I went through the motions. Next was the ultrasound room. They laid me on this table. This ultrasound tech came in all bubbly and excited, which pissed me off because I was not in the mood. Just come on and get it over with was my mindset. She took this probe straight to my armpit. I looked over to the monitor, and there was this one big white mass on the screen. She hit me with these words you never want a tech to say to you. "Let me get the doctor. I'll be right back." When I tell you, that was the longest "I'd be right back" in my life! I felt like she was gone for eight five hours. As I was in the room waiting for them to return, all I could do again was blame myself and think about my five-year-old and fifteen-year-old. Life was about to change not only for me but also for them. While the tech was gone, the tears were flowing down my face. At that moment, all I could do was cry out to my Father and ask him not to leave or forsake me. I begged God to show up in that room with me. I begged him like a child who was talking to her daddy. Father God, please spare me. Please spare my life! The doctor and the tech come back into the room. The doctor took the probe, looked around some more, and had this disturbed look on her face. Then, it hit me that we needed to get a biopsy, which needed to take place ASAP, per the physician. So they handed me a folder and scheduled me for the biopsy two days later. I looked at that folder, which was full of all the possibilities and what to expect on the day of the biopsy. My husband and I headed to the parking deck to wear another mask and face the world.

I found myself burdened with an overwhelming weight on my shoulders. I needed to inform my boss, whom I just started working for the week before, that I required an extra day off to undergo a biopsy. During the phone call, I became overwhelmed, screamed, hyperventilated, shook, and nearly vomited in my car. My boss advised me to take the day off and collect myself, but I couldn't comprehend what she said. I attempted to rationalize the situation and sat in the parking lot for two hours. Eventually, I mustered the courage to drive home. In the following days, I had to pack away my emotions and focus solely on "the investment" of being a new employee. I had to show up to work with a smile, a clear mind, and a positive attitude while dealing with my personal situation. In reality, my job was the furthest thing from my mind during that period.

Chapter FOUR

Biopsy Day

*A spiritual desert, my well has run dry, please
Lord don't pass me.*

-Dee Days

Here we are, Biopsy Day, and believe it or not, my emotional state wasn't that bad. I already knew in my heart what they were waiting to confirm. I walked in with a fighter mentality. That morning, I had a horrible attitude; I wasn't in the mood for anything or anybody. I was ready to get this over with. The nurse told me how to do this procedure and what to expect afterward. I honestly just wanted her to shut up and do it. The biopsy wasn't that bad, considering they stuck me in my breast ten individual times and underneath my arm ten more additional times. I was so sore afterward. They sent me on my way and told me I should hear something in the next two to three days.

Well, if you could imagine, those were the longest three days of my life. I felt like I had aged 30 years by the time the doctor called me. The third day came on January 17, 2023. My phone rang, and

I was at work. I ran into a patient room to take the call; ironically enough, it was room 13. Go figure! I had a seat, and she told me it was positive for cancer and it had spread to my lump nodes. Now I needed to find a breast specialist for them to go into further details as to what were the next steps. "Have a good day." She spoke to me like a factory worker. It was like it was just another run-of-the-mill phone call for her. There was no compassion in her voice. There was no empathy. It was very trivial and commercial. And boom, just like that, the call was over, and so was my life as I knew it. I had to gather myself, return to my new job, put on my mask, and make good on their investment.

Let me take a moment to lay this all out for you. I recently started a new job and still needed access to medical insurance, FMLA, or PTO because I had only been working here for a little over a week. In addition, I was a newlywed who just purchased a home with my spouse. As a mother of two boys aged five and fifteen, as well as a caregiver for an ailing elderly mother who at times requires more attention than my minor children, my plate was quite full!

Now, keep all of this in mind. I walked out of room 13, immediately clocked in, and had to help other patients when I had just become a patient myself. I went to my manager's office to tell her the news; I couldn't even get the words out of my mouth before the tears started to flow. Before I could get it out, she already knew what I would say. She attempted to be human with me, offered me some tissue, and asked if she could hug me. I was so vulnerable, weak, and emotionally drained. I was just numb; I couldn't feel anything. That moment felt like I was having an out-of-body experience; I just can't put words to describe that feeling. She allowed me to go home for the rest of the day in order to put together a game plan for the next few days. The plan was to find someone who would see me without insurance, try to get on my husband's insurance, try to make appointments, etc. At this point, I knew it was official, and IT was camping in my body, and I wanted it out now!

Results ... Xanax ... The Calls

After a few days and multiple phone calls all over Atlanta, I was able to get in with a doctor to go over the biopsy results and get official Department of Health documentation with my diagnoses on it for record-keeping. The physician came in the room, sat down, and laid it on me; she confirmed that it was cancer, and she told me, "Yea, it's pretty aggressive, and you are going to need some financial assistance to get this process started." She handed me a financial application and told me to complete it over the next few days. Someone from her office would call me to put me in a program to help with the cost of having cancer.

She gave me a prescription for Xanax and sent me on my way. All I could do at that moment was sit there and ask myself, *Did this lady just come in, tell me my life was ending, and hand me a damn application to fill out regarding money? Like, lady, that's it? Do you think I'm in the mental state to even care about some money, an application, or anything of that nature? Seriously, I have been walking around for at least two weeks, carrying this burden on me, and no one has helped me.* As I walked out of this clinic with all these resources in my hand, I looked up to the sky and said to myself, *You know what? I'm not going to "die behind some red tape." Too many women have died waiting on treatment all because they were getting shuffled around like I was.* At that moment, I became my advocate. I was so pissed with the world, and I was ready to fight. That fight or flight response had kicked in, and I was about to kick open every door until everyone listened to me and did what had to be done to get this thing out of me!

I got in my car, drove straight to my husband's job, and I told him a physician confirmed that it was cancer and that, per her, "It's aggressive." My husband pulled me out of the car, put me in his, and he went in! He started praying over me and our family. The only thing that I could say over and over was, "God, if you don't spare me for me, spare me for my babies. Spare my life for my babies. I have lived my life for me, and I have done some wrong in life, but spare my life if not for me but for my babies." Bryan continued to pray for me in his car. All I could do was rock back and forth and cry while he was praying for me. We both just sat there in silence and allowed God to move. Soon after, a calm came over the two of us, and we devised a game plan for the day. The plan was to go home, medicate myself, and rest because the next day, I had to return to my new job.

My employer started out being super supportive; they connected me with some of the best doctors. Within days, I had an appointment with a breast surgeon, a plastic surgeon, then an oncologist, an MRI, a CT scan ... you name it! One staff member even took me under her wing. She walked with me to my very first appointment with the breast specialist. She said, "I'm not going to let you walk alone; I'll sit with you until your husband gets here." With arms locked, we walked through the tunnel at our job to the other building. I said it felt like I was walking "the green mile." We both laughed and continued walking. This job was excellent, and the support was unbelievable. Oh, but that should change very soon.

Reactions And Red Tape

All of this had taken place in a matter of weeks. This tiny lump threw every hurdle you can think of at me. I had an allergic reaction to the dye they injected into me while getting the CT scan. I went into anaphylactic shock, which is a life-threatening reaction that happened quickly. It started with this itching in my nose while the dye went through my vein. Then, my throat started itching. As I was lying there, I started to clear my throat, and a few times, the tech kept telling me to lay still. After that fourth cough, she hit the red emergency button and pulled me out of the CT machine.

My face was hot, and I could feel my tongue swelling. I started pointing at my ring finger and the door to let her know I had someone with me and to go get my husband. When she saw my face, I could hear her say, "Call a code! Get EMS in here NOW!" My husband made it into the room where I was on a gurney, and he was pissed! His first reaction was, "What did y'all do to her? She was fine! What happened?" And just like that, the most crucial scan that I needed to find out if my cancer had spread could not be done. I spent a few hours in the ER, and now they have to try another way to get this scan done. Appointments got shifted around left and right, and my mother was also in and out of her doctor's appointments. One critical scan almost got canceled due to some red tape. I remember telling the scheduler that I was getting my MRI and that if I had to hold them hostage, someone was doing my scan! The scheduler laughed at me and called me crazy. She thought I was playing, which I was, but I genuinely meant every word I said to her. I was getting that scan done one way or the other.

I was not going to become a casualty behind some red tap. I had a fighter's mentality and was not about to lie down and accept whatever the doctors told me as the gospel. I had to adjust my thinking. Keep in mind that while I was juggling all of these appointments, it was time off work. That meant NO pay, and we had to pay for all those visits out of pocket. While I was knocking out visits, my husband was tackling the insurance situation. He was trying to get me on his plan during what isn't considered open enrollment for the policy.

I put all of this behind me while God went before me and prepared a place for me during this trying time. The weeks started rolling, time was ticking, and my insurance was due to kick in on March 1, 2023. The big day was March 6, 2023. Just like that, I got on my husband's insurance in the nick of time. My insurance kicked in as well. We were now preparing for the surgery, and in my thoughts, we were preparing for me never to be a whole woman again. But I was okay with this because I viewed it as becoming a better version of myself.

Boobvoyage

Before my battle with the surgeon's blade, I sought solace in the company of my dear girlfriends. Together, we celebrated life with a unique event - a "Boobvoyage" party in honor of the impending mastectomy. I knew the road ahead would be arduous, but I was determined to approach it with a lighthearted spirit. My tribe of sisters stood by me and surrounded me with love and support. We even christened the cancer with a humorous nickname and released pink balloons adorned with not-so-nice messages. As the balloons soared skywards, so did my spirits, and the cancer receded, powerless against the strength of our bond. In that moment, I found a sense of peace. An emotional calm soothed my soul. My dear friends gifted me with items I would need for the journey ahead, and their love and support kept me strong.

I decided to do something like this to make my battle feel okay to me. It was like a form of therapy. The girls showered me with post-surgery gifts. A few girls encouraged me, and prayers were spoken over me. Overall, it was a beautiful day. I felt prepared to have my breast removed now. I was on an emotional high. But when the days were over, this tiny voice in the back of my mind kept whispering, *I was not going to be a whole woman again.* As the hour of my surgery drew near, my very essence felt poised to crumble like pillars of a once-great temple. My breasts, my hair, my femininity - all were to be stripped away, leaving me bare and vulnerable. The days leading up to the fateful moment were a tempestuous whirlwind of emotions that tossed me here and there. My every waking moment was consumed with preparations as I attended a flurry of appointments with specialists in breast health, plastic surgery, and oncology. The sands of time seemed to blur and bleed together, and each day spilled into the next. My body and mind were exhausted. I struggled to comprehend what lay ahead, and the moments slipped past me like sand through my fingers. Fading moments and memories seemed impossible to hold onto.

As a family, we were uncertain about what the next three months would entail. As we approached the surgery weekend, I felt it was essential to spend some quality time alone with Bryan while I was still whole and complete. But parenting called, and we couldn't get our time in. I was very disappointed, but when you are a parent, that always trumps what you have going on. Responsibilities continue even when it comes to having this thing called cancer. Again, it isn't cute, and I don't care! Life continued, and I knew I better get on the train, or it would pass me by. There was no time for whimpering and weakness. The way my life was set up, I couldn't be weak. A serene calm enveloped me on the morning of the surgery, and my mind was at peace. The only thing on my mind was the urgency to remove the cancer from my body. Losing my breast was not a concern at the time; I was just relieved to rid myself of this disease. As we waited in the waiting room, Bryan, Brittney, Mel, and Ivy prayed for my safety and gathered around me. Their warm embraces steadied my nerves as I entered the surgery preparation room. Before I left, I entrusted Brittney with a letter I had written to Bryan. It would be given to him only after I had gone under the knife. I wanted him to feel my presence even when I was away, and the letter expressed my immense love and gratitude for his unwavering support during this challenging time in our marriage.

Awakenings

It was a four-and-a-half-hour surgery. When I woke up from surgery, Bryan and Brittney were there. The first thing I did was place my hands on my chest to see how much of my breast did they leave me. When I looked down at them, I first said, "Oh, that's where they're supposed to be." Everyone in the room laughed and shook their heads. So, to my surprise, I also received a breast lift. Which I guess you could say was a plus. A haze was still around me days after I got home from the hospital. Things were in slow motion; Bryan handled Brayden and Bryce for me. My phone wasn't ringing that much. Life was on pause. And sadly enough, I had to have my breast removed to get some reprieve from the world. Oddly, that was the way my life was set up.

Like most women, we run, manage, organize everything for everybody, and neglect ourselves. Again, honestly, that was why I was in that situation. During my recovery, I spent a lot of days praying, coloring for anxiety, looking out the window, and journaling. Overall, I spent time with myself and tried to adapt to my new norm. I promised myself that my boys wouldn't see me lying in bed when they got home from school every day. The things that we do as moms to protect our kids. I forced myself downstairs every day around two-thirty and sat in the living room. My baby boy would always like to climb onto my lap and cuddle. Still, of course, during the recovery, I had several bandages and four drain tubs coming from my chest. So, I came up with this story that Mommy had surgery on her arm, and that's why you can't lay on me. Luckily, he bought it, and we rolled with that. The crazy thing about this cancer walk and what they don't tell you to prepare you for is how even while trying to adjust, recover, and heal, you still have to protect those around you who aren't emotionally mature enough to handle the pressures of cancer treatment.

A few weeks into recovering, I went in to have my port placed. On the morning of that surgery, I was being ridiculous. I felt like the port placement was the start of the fight process. I imagined myself standing in the corner of my boxing ring; the other corner was cancer. As they were preparing to take me into surgery, I had Bryan turn on the ROCKY theme Song "Eye of the Tiger," I put my fist up and said, "Baby, I'll be back. We are getting ready to fight. And in typical Bryan fashion, he just looked at me, smiled, and shook his head. Making light of the situation helped me cope with what was happening; it gave me a lighter perspective. Because I genuinely feel like your attitude and mindset enable you to overcome tough times.

Chapter FIVE

The Red Devil

When the devil comes at you, maybe you are trying to do something right.

-Denzel Washington

During the first three months of recovery, I found emotional, physical, and mental solace, which prepared me for chemotherapy. When I took my first tour of the chemotherapy room, I couldn't complete the walk-through. It was the longest hallway I had ever walked down, and upon reaching the end, the room opened up with bright lights and windows all around. Overcome with fear, I saw a room full of people who appeared to be half-dead, wrapped in blankets, and barely awake. This sight was too much to bear, given that I was about to join their ranks. I immediately turned to Bryan, buried my head into his chest, and then had to leave the room.

Doxorubicin (The Red Devil)

Over the next few days, I started preparing myself for Chemo Day. I was nervous and anxious because I was ready to start, so it could soon be over. Chemo started on April 20th. I first started on the most aggressive form of chemo, Doxorubicin (The Red Devil). It has this nickname because of its color and severe side effects. At four hours long, this was the most grueling appointment I had ever endured.

This massive treatment room had reclining chairs, lighting, open windows, and at least 20 to 30 people. Each person had a caregiver to sit with them as they received treatment. People brought books, snacks, puzzles, or a mobile device to distract them from what was happening. I always wanted to sit near the window, look out, and absorb the moment of what was happening to me. I couldn't believe that this was what my life had become. I'd always taken care of people. I was never a person to be taken care of! All I could do was sit there and watch this poisonous drug drip by drip as it slowly entered my body. The physician told me that it could potentially cause damage to my heart, kidney, and liver. All I could do was just pray that this drug that was killing the cancer wouldn't kill me as well.

I made it through the first round of treatment. I was so tired, hurt, disgusted, disappointed, and drugged up. All I could do was go home and climb in the bed that day. I slept for five hours straight. My kids came home that evening, and I had to find some way to act like everything was normal. *Mommy was her typical self, and things were good.* Again, I had to put on an act to protect my kids. At that time, I felt like no one was protecting me. About fourteen days into the Doxorubicin "Red Devil," I wouldn't allow the nurses to call it that when they would verify the drug. I told them you are not putting anything into me that's referred to as a DEVIL! I told them if it had a nickname, we would call it the blood of JESUS! They looked at me like *okay, lady, whatever.* I just refused to have something that was going into my body called the "devil" around me. Hence, as the treatment went on every two weeks or so, the side effects started to kick in quickly.

Hair Today ... GONE Tomorrow

Before my dance with the Red Devil, I made a bold move and decided to chop off my hair. It was the one thing I had control over during this chaos. I couldn't bear to watch it fall out in clumps, so I called up my ride-or-die friend, Shanta. She was a total champ and even untied my hair for me - perhaps for the last time. We laughed, and I felt empowered to take on this new phase.

I asked Shanta if she remembered back in the day when girls were about to get into a fight; they would tie their hair back so the other girl couldn't pull it. She said, "YES!" I said, "Well, I cut mine off, so while I'm in this fight, she (cancer) won't have anything to grab hold of. We both laughed as the barber commenced to cut off my hair. She gave me a low buzz cut to start with. The barber didn't want to make me completely ball. She was optimistic by saying maybe it wouldn't come out totally. After my haircut appointment, I went home with my baby boy Bryce, who met me there. As he approached me and looked at my head, he started to cry. He said that I looked like a boy and wanted my old brown hair back. Suddenly he ran off. That hurt me badly, and I felt like a monster. My baby didn't even think I was pretty anymore. OMG, God, how am I going to do this? My baby is afraid of me and thinks I look like a boy.

Again, "Cancer ain't cute, and this is what they don't tell you." About two weeks after treatment, my hair started to come out in clumps. It only took a few more days of drastic hair loss to cement my decision to shave it off and go completely bald. I had my "newfound" friend/coworker shave it off for me. I couldn't even face the mirror the night she shaved it off in my bathroom. I sat in a chair with my back turned to the mirror. When she was done, all I could do was cry because I watched what I thought made me beautiful get taken away. She (Cancer) took my beauty, and I was mad at her. It made me want to fight her, and I was ready. She took everything from me, and I wanted my shit back! In my mind, cancer was a person who had come into my life. She took my beauty. She tried to take my life. She took my money and tried to take my man and my friends. When someone comes in and takes your things, what would you do? You fight! From that moment on, I made up my mind; I was in fight mode.

For weeks, I couldn't look at myself. I would take showers in the dark and turn my back to the mirror when I would get out of the shower. I soon got over that and reminded myself that I was fighting a thing that had come in and taken my stuff. I would tell myself. *Girl, get it together, get your shit back.* When I was sick or tired, I gave myself these words of affirmation.

Radiated

Radiation fibrosis is a devastating condition that can cause persistent pain, stiffness, tightness, and hardening of the breast and surrounding torso area. The condition is caused by radiation therapy and can last for a lifetime. The affected area becomes hardened, making moving difficult and causing severe discomfort. The rib area is particularly vulnerable to the condition because, in breast cancer, the radiation usually affects the rib area as well. Despite the best efforts of medical professionals, there is no known cure for this condition, and the symptoms may never entirely go away.

In radiation fibrosis, you develop a massive amount of scar tissue, a limited range of motion, and swelling where your breast has been radiated. It feels like a cinder block is resting on your chest. Your breasts are tight and shrunken. Shockingly, you can't lay on that side. It's uncomfortable. I slept with multiple pillows propped underneath and around me every night. I couldn't even comfortably lay next to my husband due to the pain that I was enduring on my left side, where my radiation took place. I had to attend physical therapy to regain the range of motion on that side. Lifting my arm past my ear, oh yeah, that was a NO! I couldn't even reach my arm behind my back to either wash or scratch it. That was what radiation did to me.

But again, I say cancer ain't cute, and this is what they don't tell you.

Underneath the clothes were several areas of my body that had third-degree burns. The burns were on my breast, underneath my arm, back, torso area, and chest just below my collarbone. There would be times when I would remove my uniform, and pieces of my skin would fall off and hit the ground; there were even times when my skin would be in my chair at work. I would be so embarrassed and ashamed. I would hurry to grab the pieces of my skin, wrap it up in a tissue, and throw it away before anyone could see. However, I managed to continue to work every day during radiation. I would have a trusted coworker come in and wrap my chest with gauze and tape so as not to irritate my skin while I was working. My skin was so sensitive the clothes would make tiny pieces fall off. It was raw and red, and several open wounds oozed fluid at times. The wounds were so bad that I was prescribed an antibiotic cream that had to be applied to prevent any infections. The thing that hurt the most was while I was enduring this gut-wrenching pain, I felt alone. Where was my support, everybody? Where were they? My body was not the body I'd been accustomed to for 42 years. How had this all become my new norm? It was as if I'd been born again but as a different version of my original self.

I continued to push through. I continued to smile through my pain and when asked, "Are you OK?" "Why are you walking like that, or why are you looking like that? What's wrong with you?" One day, I had to tell someone, "Don't ask me what's wrong with me anymore." I swear I wanted to cuss her out for that insensitive question. You should be good now you're done with chemo, but what people fail to realize is that radiation is a beast all of its own. Radiation is like the redheaded stepchild that nobody talks about, and people treated me as such. People acted like, *Oh, it's just radiation. They're not pumping you with poison anymore.* But, what people failed to realize was that although they were not pumping me with poison anymore, they were burning me from the inside out. The lack of empathy during my radiation stage was so painful, mentally and emotionally. I fell into a very dark, deep depression. However, I want you to remember I'm a mom of two active boys. So I had no time to stay depressed very long.

I'm a wife, and I'm a daughter. I'm a caregiver. I'm a mom. There were times that I couldn't even be a patient, and there were times I couldn't even be sick! It would upset me to know that so many people depended on me that I couldn't even just BE. I would always tell my husband I can't even have cancer in peace! So, what I decided to do once the circus surrounding me having cancer had died down was to dig myself out of this mess. I was not only determined to be mom, daughter, friend, and wife, but I was doing things differently. I made it a priority to say, "No, this is my time, this is my day, and I will rest. I will feel. I will be sick. I will be happy; I permit myself to be whatever I want and do not seek permission."

Mommy Duties / Precautions

My son Bryce's 6th birthday took place the day after my first treatment. We had planned to celebrate his belated birthday party two days after his birthday. Everyone told me I was crazy for going through with the party. Even Bryan thought I was ridiculous, but I worked hard to stay present as a mom for my boys.

I didn't care because, in my mind, I didn't know if this would be my last birthday with my baby boy. No one explores all of the emotional challenges you may be faced with when you get diagnosed with cancer, and no one thinks about the toll it takes on raising kids while going through treatment. This isn't considered the normal part of a cancer journey, but it is! We are still mothers and daughters and wives. We're still all of the things we were before becoming a cancer patient. How did I push through the party? I had a lot of help from friends to get me through the day. The support system that I have always relied on throughout my life, my mother, still required my assistance during this period. I found myself in an unfamiliar position, unsure how to balance caring for her and caring for myself.

Chemo is an extremely powerful and dangerous treatment. Come to find out, it is so powerful that it can be passed on to your partner. So therefore, one of the many precautions is that after chemo, you must abstain from all physical contact for seventy hours to protect others. They call this your shedding period because the chemo comes out of your body through sweat, tears, bowel, urine, saliva, and other body secretions. So, we did a few things to ensure that everyone was safe in the house. We quarantined my bathroom, and no one could use it. I slept on an air mattress in my bedroom next to my bed. My husband would have become sick because the meds made me sweat a lot at night. Sweat-to-skin contact could transfer the chemo to others. Whenever I sweated a lot, I wouldn't allow my kids to hug me. Can you imagine the unbearable level of loneliness and depression that I felt during this time? The little hair I had was coming out in clumps; my breasts and taste buds were gone. It tasted like I had a sack of nickels in my mouth. To top it off, my mother was sick in the hospital, and our bank account was getting low!

Chapter SIX

Can A Sista Get A Break?

My grace is sufficient for you, for my power is made perfect in weakness.

-2 Corinthians 12:9-10

It seemed as though every aspect of my life was under attack, and I was struggling to make sense of it all. However, I failed to recognize that this was divine intervention at work, and it molded me into a stronger, more faithful person. It took losing everything to reveal where my true source of strength lay.

Mama!

As I approached the end of my first two sets of chemo, I got a call that my mother's condition had drastically worsened, and I needed to get to her NOW. I asked the nurse how much longer I had on the machine, and she told me that I had about an hour left. I also needed to see my physician after this appointment because I was having an issue with my port. I was in a panic! I needed to get to my mother to get her to the ER! I asked the nurse if she could speed up the machine's drip so I could get out of there sooner. She asked the Dr, and he thought I was crazy! I told them I WAS going crazy sitting here worrying about my mother. So here I go again, putting others before my situation. He allowed the nurse to speed the drip up, and I told the Dr. I would send a picture of my port. I gotta go! Although I was high on Benadryl, dizzy, nauseous, and had diarrhea, I took Mom to the ER. OMG, I had to make two bathroom stops before we even got to the hospital.

After fourteen hours in the ER, Mom finally got admitted into the hospital, and with me having no other assistants with her, I was not about to leave my mother. For four days, I stayed right there by her side, and I'd do it again. I was dealing with the side effects of the most aggressive form of chemo a person with breast cancer can take. I was two weeks out from returning back to work after my leave of absence and still struggling to "recover" from a double mastectomy and four weeks of chemo. And I turned around and got sick with some virus while being in the hospital with my mother. All I could say was, are you kidding me? Life ... really?

Again, "Cancer ain't cute; this is what they don't tell you." Those sixteen rounds / six months of chemo and five weeks of radiation were physically painful, mentally draining, and emotionally scary! While still trying to work during this time, I had numerous setbacks, doctor appointments, and several trips to the ER for myself and my mom. Keep in mind now that I am her caregiver as well. At the same time, I was trying to maintain my sanity and hold down a job. All of this made me a complicated person to deal with because I felt as if no one understood what I was going through. I felt like life kept piling up on me, and no one was there to take the pressure off me. I can't imagine how this affected the people around me. Despite mood swings, tears, and complaints, my friends never failed to answer the phone when I called. They always provided a safe space to let me vent about everything.

Setbacks? You Should Be Good Now?

Radiation therapy was a time-consuming and challenging process that demanded significant patience, perseverance, and endurance. The treatment entailed daily sessions that lasted up to five or six weeks while I attempted to maintain other obligations, such as work schedules. Unfortunately, during my radiation treatment, I experienced several major setbacks that made the process even more challenging, including developing bacterial pneumonia and testing positive for pregnancy due to hormonal fluctuations. These complications necessitated additional testing and time away from treatment. Worrying about the potential growth of any cancer in my body made my anxiety levels soar! By the time I received clearance to resume radiation therapy, I had already missed four treatments. Two sessions daily, six hours apart, were required in order to catch up. This schedule adversely affected my work schedule, finances, and ability to support my husband, who had to take on additional work shifts.

By now it seemed that the sympathy and empathy have gone out of the window. Because you're at what most think is the end of treatment, you "should be good now." Oh, you have no idea how much that used to piss me off! I wanted to scream at the top of my lungs. What in your mind would make you think I'm good now? I'm sitting here working with third-degree burns under my arm, my chest, and my torso. NO, I AM NOT GOOD!

It's impossible to downplay the weight of loneliness, and its overwhelming presence consumed me. My anger and frustration with life left me feeling joyless. However, when confronted with such crucial moments in life, it's essential to focus on self-care and avoid external distractions that might derail the process.

Maintaining balance amid life's challenges was an ongoing struggle, and illness only exacerbated the difficulties. Nevertheless, I had to find the strength to persevere, knowing that the work of healing and recovery was entirely on me. It's disheartening how normalized a cancer diagnosis has become. There's nothing commercial about battling this disease, and yet, society seems to be insensitive to the overwhelming challenges we face. It's disheartening to witness how people perceive cancer as if it's a common cold. Why would anyone downplay the severity of such a serious illness?

It's so distasteful how people leverage our struggles with cancer for commercial gain. It's used as a marketing tool to promote their products. True cancer awareness is not about donning a ribbon, pink tutu, or t-shirt. Rather, it's about bringing attention to the harsh reality of the disease and dispelling the notion that it's some attractive or glamorous social club. It's essential to acknowledge the dismissive and insensitive attitudes that cancer patients often encounter when people think and say ...

"We're good now."

Proper cancer awareness should include educating people on how to communicate with and treat cancer patients after treatment is over. During my experience, I've heard some really insensitive statements and received gifts intended to uplift but failed. It's essential to bring awareness and educate people on what's appropriate. Here are a few things that I encountered and what I did to counter these statements in my mind and heart:

"But you're okay now, right?"

It's natural to feel like things won't be okay anymore, given the hardships one endures during and after a challenging treatment. However, we must remember that we are stronger from fighting those struggles, and things will improve. We might be better than before since we have faced adversity and emerged victorious. Consequently, life may seem a little sweeter now.

"I don't know how you do it!"

I'm choosing to fight over dying. Yeah, that's a no-brainer; hello? We have to trust in the Lord and hope for the best.

"You got this!"

Really, you have cancer? You don't look that sick."

Really, what the hell does sick look like?

"My _____ died of cancer."

Look, I get it. All of the comments are made to emphasize

the shared experience of battling cancer. However, every individual's cancer journey is unique and personal. And we don't wanna hear how someone has died. This tactic is completely counter-productive

Indeed, most people often lack the knowledge of what to say or avoid saying anything to someone fighting cancer. Still, I also believe the root issue is a complete lack of empathy. Cancer awareness programs should prioritize empathy and awareness rather than merely superficial displays of support like pink ribbons or shirts.

"Or girl, why are you tripping? Your about to get some new boobs."

I don't think people realize how this sounds. There is nothing new about having something amputated from your body resulting in never having feelings in that part of your body. There is nothing NEW or FUN about that!

I'm not getting some free boob job. Would you tell a person who just had their leg cut off? Well, hey, look at it this way. On the bright side, you only have to buy one shoe now. Or, what would you say to a person who has to go on dialysis? Well, at least you don't have to worry about going to pee anymore. The machine will do it for you.

"You're going to be fine."

This statement used to infuriate me whenever someone said it to me. It made me feel like my struggles were not significant enough to be taken seriously. It was almost as if the person was saying, "Come on, just get over it already." Don't tell me everything will be fine; it's not fine! People need to understand that healing is not a quick process, and I cannot simply snap out of it. It's a long journey that will continue for the rest of my life. Feeling fine is something I will have to strive for every day.

"Stay Positive."

I can't believe it! When you hear that your life may be in danger, it's hard to stay positive. Society needs to be more aware of how their words can impact others. Instead of telling someone to be positive, it's better not to say anything if you have nothing good to say.

Saying, *"At least you caught it early."*

It can feel like a slap in the face. What if there was no early? What if I didn't have it at all? These are things to consider when supporting someone in a difficult situation.

"Congrats, your treatment is over!"

Yes, the chemo or radiation part is over, but more work still needs to be done. Is my cancer gone? What happens next? How will the new meds they have me on affect me now? What does life look like for me now and can cancer come back?

What happened to all the support I had when going through chemo? I still need support more than ever before. Mentally, we still need the occasional check-ins. We still need to know that people care. People need to know that just because I'm not sitting in a chemo chair every week or lying on a cold radiation table, I still have fears and anxiety looming in the back of my head. Any time I feel a slight lump or bump anywhere in my body, I worry it is cancer. And I have no one to call late at night discuss it with because people feel like, *Ok, it's been a year. Get over it, or oh god, girl, are you still worried about that?*

Awareness, in my opinion, needs to be when people are made aware of how they need to be sensitive to this thing called cancer and that it goes beyond what mainstream media shows you. It goes beyond chemo and radiation. Years after treatment, our bodies are still recovering, and we walk around praying that the medicines that we took to stay alive haven't damaged other organs in our bodies.

Help ... Support Needed

Webster's dictionary defines AWARE as vigilance in observing or alertness in drawing inferences from what one experiences. Proper awareness involves being a compassionate and empathetic person who is in tune with the needs of their loved ones. It means being there for them during their initial diagnosis or treatment and especially after the initial attention has faded. To truly understand someone, you need to know what brings them joy and happiness and be mindful of what makes them tick. It helps if you are attentive to their needs and willing to lend a helping hand whenever they require it. Proper awareness is not just about being present; it is about fully engaging with the people you care about and doing everything you can to improve their lives.

After the difficult time was over, what I needed was for my friends and family to stay in touch with me. "I longed for my family and friends to see me as a person who was still recovering. I yearned for them to understand that despite my best efforts, I was not invincible, and I needed their help to make it through each day. Although they often complimented me on how well I was doing, I still required special attention and care during my recovery process. I couldn't help but feel responsible for this because I tried to put up a facade of normalcy to my loved ones. Concealing my pain and need for emotional support may not have been the right move. It was a challenging and isolating experience, but I remained hopeful that one day, I would heal and no longer need to hide my vulnerabilities. I needed them to be patient and understand that constantly talking about my illness was only sometimes helpful. Sometimes, just having a normal conversation about nothing was the best support I could receive. We were living with the situation every day, and talking about it all the time was exhausting.

I needed people to help me break out of my routine. Something as simple as walking with a friend, grabbing a smoothie, or having lunch would have been nice. These activities would have helped me get moving again. It would have been especially helpful if people who knew my likes and what makes me happy took the time to do those little things with me. Early on, having those supporters would have made a huge difference. After completing my treatment, I was eagerly expecting to receive support and love from my family and friends, but unfortunately, I didn't get any. It was a harsh reality for me, but I learned to find peace in solitude and started relying on myself for inner peace, which has been an ongoing battle for me to this day. I came to realize that in life, people come and go like seasons, and while it would be great to have constant support, it's not always possible. However, the only thing that remains consistent is my faith in myself and God, who I know will never abandon me. The universe prepared me to be strong, and I had no choice but to be strong. My mother was ill, my husband was working non-stop, and I was in a new job that required me to learn quickly. Everything that could have made me weak was taken away, and I had to push through if I wanted to survive. A life-altering situation taught me to be resilient, independent, and self-reliant. Even though it was a challenging process, I learned to embrace and grow from it.

Chapter SEVEN

A New Normal Nobody Asked For!

If there is no struggle, there is no progress

-Frederick Douglass

Life is unpredictable, and for those of us battling cancer, it can be a particularly tumultuous journey. We approach this challenge with determination and resilience. However, while undergoing treatment, it can be challenging to navigate daily life, whether at work or school. A little empathy and understanding can make a significant difference. Kindness and consideration are vital to those of us fighting this battle.

Adjusting to life after treatment and seeking a new normal can be challenging. It can be difficult to determine what the new normal is. In addition, there may be permanent scars on the body, which can lead to a sense of uncertainty. It's crucial to prioritize follow-up care, manage side effects, and care for yourself and others. Even after treatment, lingering side effects can persist. Acknowledging that the body and spirit may sometimes feel exhausted is essential. Relaxing and focusing on self-care is crucial to healing and finding a new sense of normalcy.

This journey of fighting cancer will last a lifetime. I have learned that despite being dealt a difficult hand, I must continue to live with the determination to fight and survive. For me, this means facing this challenge head-on. I cannot allow myself to be weak or surround myself with those who pity me. I am a warrior, a fighter, a mother, a woman, a friend, and a wife. Through this experience, I have discovered an internal power and strength I never knew existed. Cancer has shown me that I am stronger than I ever imagined. It has allowed me to start again and to begin a new chapter in my life. While it may seem counterintuitive, God had to stop me to start me all over again. I hope this book will inspire other women facing similar challenges. Pause, reflect, and allow God to stop and start you all over again on the journey of self-discovery and renewal.

Whatever your motivation is to live, whether it be your children, cat, dog, friends, mother, or spouse, I encourage you to put your blinders on and focus on that one thing. Let that one thing motivate you to fight, endure the suffering, and get to the other end. Touch that one thing that drove you to put force and power behind you. Embrace every round of chemo or radiation. Know that with each treatment, you are one step closer to taking back control of your life. Don't be discouraged. Don't be dismayed and face the battle head-on.

Look forward to it.

Look forward to the hair loss, the pain, the fatigue, and the body aches. Fight and keep going. Know you will get to the end and be restored. You will receive blessings from the Lord because that's His word. Suffering may endure for a night, but joy comes in the morning!

My story continues ...

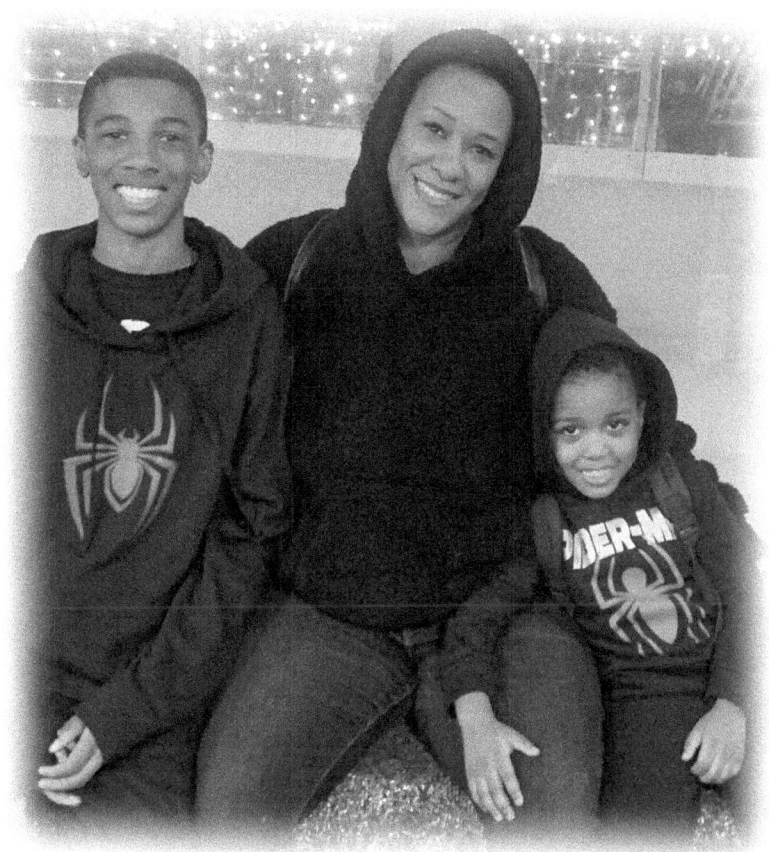

A Letter to My Boys

Life can be tough, and we will never get it all right, but I hope both of you saw your mom as a strong woman who never gave up, no matter what obstacles I faced. I fought hard and loved fiercely. I didn't have much to give, but what I gave to the two of you was the greatest part of me and the greatest commandment of all: LOVE!

"A mother is the son's first true love; a son is their mother's last true love."

~Love Mommy

www.ingramcontent.com/pod-product-compliance
Lightning Source LLC
Chambersburg PA
CBHW051649120626
46551CB00015B/2275